I0774660

COMPLETE GUIDE TO UNDERSTANDING GASTROSCOPY

Essential Techniques, Procedures, Best Practices For Accurate Diagnosis And Effective Treatment

KLEIN HOYLE

© [KLEIN HOYLE] [2024]

All rights reserved.

No part of this book may be reproduced, distributed, or transmitted in any form or by any means, including photocopying, recording, or other electronic or mechanical methods, without the publisher's prior written permission, with the exception of brief quotations in critical reviews and certain other noncommercial uses permitted by copyright law.

Disclaimer

The content in this book is based on the author's expertise and comprehension of the topic. The author has no affiliation or link with any corporation, business, or person. This book is meant to give general information and educational material only, and it should not be interpreted as professional medical advice. Always seek the advice of a skilled healthcare expert if you have any queries about medical issues or treatments. The author and publisher expressly disclaim any responsibility resulting directly or indirectly from the use or use of the information included in this book.

Table of Contents

ABOUT THIS BOOK

The "Complete Guide to Understanding Gastroscopy" is an invaluable resource for both healthcare professionals and patients, providing detailed insights into the complexities of this critical diagnostic technique. From its fundamental principles to cutting-edge developments, each chapter looks into critical areas that lead to a comprehensive grasp of gastroscopy and its ramifications.

Beginning with Chapter 1, readers are introduced to the principles of gastroscopy and its role in contemporary healthcare. This section delves into the complexities of the gastrointestinal system and explains the critical function of gastroscopy in diagnosis, establishing the groundwork for further investigation.

Chapter 2 offers vital advice on preparing for a gastroscopy, including food limitations, medication regimes, and mental preparation recommendations.

This proactive strategy assures optimum patient preparedness, which improves the procedure's effectiveness and safety.

Moving on, Chapter 3 provides a detailed analysis of the gastroscopy technique, including step-by-step instructions, the function of endoscopes, anesthetic alternatives, and possible hazards. By demystifying the operation, patients may approach it with confidence, while healthcare providers gain insights into how to improve patient outcomes.

In Chapter 4, readers are taken inside the gastroscopy suite, where they learn about the endoscopy room, the equipment used, and the critical duties of healthcare personnel. This section focuses on patient comfort measurements and emphasizes the necessity of a supportive atmosphere conducive to the best results.

Chapter 5 focuses on the patient's trip, with careful information provided on everything from arrival to post-procedure care.

This chapter encourages empathy and understanding by revealing the patient experience, both of which are critical components of providing patient-centered care.

Chapter 6 looks into analyzing gastroscopy data, enabling readers to evaluate discoveries, comprehend typical problems discovered, and determine the importance of biopsy samples. Effective communication tactics keep patients informed and involved throughout their healthcare experience.

Safety is crucial, as shown in Chapter 7, which exhaustively details possible difficulties, emergency procedures, and safety regulations. Healthcare practitioners foster trust and responsibility by protecting patients' rights and fighting for their well-being.

Chapter 8 focuses on post-procedure care and lifestyle suggestions, stressing the significance of follow-up visits and close monitoring.

This section promotes long-term health and well-being by encouraging patients to take proactive actions.

Special populations need adapted techniques, as discussed in Chapter 9, which covers gastroscopy in youngsters, the elderly, pregnant women, and patients with particular medical disorders. Healthcare practitioners promote fair access to excellent treatment by tailoring procedures to the requirements of individual patients.

Finally, Chapter 10 looks forward to the future of gastroscopy, noting rising technology, research opportunities, and the procedure's increasing role in healthcare. By embracing innovation and ongoing development, the medical community can stay at the forefront of diagnostic excellence.

CHAPTER 1

Introduction To Gastroscopy

What Is Gastroscopy?

Gastroscopy is a medical treatment that examines the upper gastrointestinal system, which includes the esophagus, stomach, and duodenum. It requires the use of a gastroscope, a thin, flexible tube with a small camera and light connected to it. The gastroscope is placed into the mouth and then directed down the throat to the stomach and duodenum.

During the process, the gastroscope's camera feeds pictures to a display, enabling the healthcare professional to study the upper digestive system lining in real-time. This allows for the identification of any anomalies, such as inflammation, ulcers, tumors, or other digestive-related problems.

Why Is A Gastroscopy Performed?

Gastroscopy is done for a variety of reasons, the most common being diagnostic and therapeutic. It is often used to look into symptoms including prolonged abdomen discomfort, trouble swallowing, heartburn, vomiting blood, unexplained weight loss, or anemia. It may also be used to screen for specific illnesses, such as esophageal cancer, or to track the course of an existing gastrointestinal ailment.

The method is also useful for collecting tissue samples (biopsies) for further examination. Biopsies may be used to diagnose illnesses such as gastritis, Helicobacter pylori infection, celiac disease, and malignancy. Gastroscopy may be coupled with other procedures, such as endoscopic ultrasonography or endoscopic retrograde cholangiopancreatography (ERCP), to provide a more thorough examination.

Overview Of The GI Tract

Understanding the architecture of the gastrointestinal (GI) tract is critical for grasping the scope of gastroscopy. The gastrointestinal tract (GI) is a long, hollow tube that starts at the mouth and terminates at the anus. It is responsible for food digestion and absorption and is made up of various parts, including the esophagus, stomach, small intestine, and large intestine.

The esophagus is a muscular tube that links the pharynx and stomach. Its major purpose is to transfer ingested food and liquids from the mouth to the stomach via a sequence of synchronized muscular spasms known as peristalsis. The stomach is a J-shaped structure in the upper belly that uses gastric fluids to partly digest food before transferring it into the small intestine.

The small intestine is the longest component of the gastrointestinal system and is separated into three sections: the duodenum, jejunum, and ileum. It is essential for the absorption of nutrients from digested foods into the circulation. The large intestine, often known as the colon, collects water and electrolytes from undigested food and produces excrement for disposal.

The Role Of Gastroscopy In Diagnosis

Gastroscopy is an effective diagnostic procedure for detecting a variety of gastrointestinal problems and illnesses. By offering a direct view of the upper digestive system, healthcare personnel may spot anomalies that other diagnostic procedures, such as X-rays or blood tests, may not reveal.

One of the most notable benefits of gastroscopy is its capacity to identify early indicators of cancer or pre-cancerous disorders in the esophagus, stomach, and duodenum. Early identification of gastrointestinal cancers is critical for enhancing treatment results and prognosis.

Furthermore, gastroscopy may detect peptic ulcers, gastroesophageal reflux disease (GERD), Barrett's esophagus, esophagitis, gastritis, and hiatal hernia. It also plays an important role in the treatment of these disorders, directing treatments such as polyp removal, stricture dilatation, and stent implantation to remove blockages.

Overall, gastroscopy gives essential information on the health and function of the upper gastrointestinal tract, which aids in the diagnosis and treatment of a variety of digestive illnesses and diseases.

CHAPTER 2

Preparing For Gastroscopy

Dietary Restriction Before The Procedure

Before conducting a gastroscopy, it is essential to adhere to specified dietary restrictions to guarantee accurate results and limit the risk of problems during the surgery. Typically, patients are instructed not to eat or drink anything for some time before their evaluation. This fasting time ensures that the stomach is empty, allowing for clearer sight of the gastrointestinal system throughout the process.

It is critical that you strictly adhere to your healthcare provider's fasting recommendations. Patients are often urged not to eat or drink for at least six to eight hours before the gastroscopy. This includes solid meals, drinks, and chewing gum. Adherence to these instructions is critical to reducing the risk of aspiration, which occurs when food or liquid enters the lungs during the surgery and leads to problems such as pneumonia.

In rare situations, your healthcare professional may give you special instructions for taking particular drugs before the surgery. To get the greatest results, please follow these directions. Additionally, if you have any questions or concerns regarding dietary limitations before your gastroscopy, please address them with your healthcare professional.

Medication Guidelines

Before having a gastroscopy, it is important to discuss your drug routine with your healthcare physician. Some drugs may need to be changed or temporarily discontinued before the surgery to lower the risk of problems and ensure accurate findings.

Nonsteroidal anti-inflammatory medicines (NSAIDs), such as ibuprofen and aspirin, may need to be discontinued several days before the gastroscopy due to an increased risk of bleeding during the operation. Furthermore, blood thinners such as warfarin or clopidogrel may need to be altered or temporarily discontinued to limit the risk of excessive bleeding during the gastroscopy.

It is important to tell your doctor about any medicines you are taking, including prescriptions, over-the-counter meds, and vitamins. Your healthcare practitioner will offer particular advice depending on your medical history and current medicines.

In rare situations, your doctor may prescribe drugs to help you relax or alleviate pain during the gastroscopy. These drugs are usually given soon before the treatment and may be taken orally or by IV. It is critical that you carefully follow your healthcare provider's recommendations while using these drugs.

What To Expect During The Pre-Procedure Assessment

Before having a gastroscopy, you will usually have a pre-procedure consultation with your doctor or a member of the medical team. During this examination, your healthcare professional will go over your medical history, present symptoms, and any medicines you are taking.

Your healthcare professional may also do a physical examination to examine your general health and identify any risk factors that may impact the treatment. This may entail monitoring your vital indicators, such as blood pressure, heart rate, and temperature.

In rare situations, your doctor may request further tests or imaging examinations to assess your gastrointestinal system further. These procedures might include blood testing, imaging investigations like X-rays or CT scans, or other specialist tests to check the health of your digestive system.

During the pre-operation examination, you should talk honestly with your healthcare practitioner and express any questions you have concerning the gastroscopy surgery. Your healthcare professional will explain what to anticipate during the process, including any possible risks or consequences, and will answer any questions you may have.

Mental Preparation Tips

Some people find it difficult or anxiety-inducing to undergo any medical treatment, even a gastroscopy. However, there are a few mental preparation suggestions that might help you feel more at ease and calm before the treatment.

First, you must educate yourself on the gastroscopy process. Understanding what to anticipate throughout the operation, including the preparatory process, the equipment used, and what happens afterward, might assist in reducing fear and uncertainty.

Furthermore, relaxation methods such as deep breathing exercises, meditation, or visualization may assist decrease anxiety and increase tranquility before the gastroscopy. These approaches may be used in the days leading up to the operation and just before the appointment.

Discuss any worries or anxieties you have regarding the gastroscopy surgery with your healthcare physician or a member of the medical team. They can reassure you, answer any concerns you may have, and provide more assistance or resources as required.

Finally, bringing a support person with you to the visit might give comfort and emotional support throughout the gastroscopy process. Having someone you know at your side might help alleviate anxiety and give confidence during the procedure.

CHAPTER 3

Understanding The Gastroscopy Procedure

A Step-By-Step Overview Of Gastroscopy

Gastroscopy is a technique performed by physicians to inspect the interior of your upper digestive tract. It's an essential tool for detecting and treating a variety of gastrointestinal disorders. Here's a step-by-step explanation of what occurs during a gastroscopy:

1. Preparing for the Procedure: Before the gastroscopy, your doctor will give you advice on how to prepare. This may entail fasting for a certain length of time to ensure your stomach is empty. It is critical to carefully follow these directions to get accurate results and reduce dangers.

2. Checking Vital Signs: When you come for the treatment, the medical personnel will take your vital signs, including blood pressure, heart rate, and oxygen level. They will also inquire about any allergies, medical problems, and drugs you are taking.

3. Anesthetic: Depending on the facility and your preferences, you may be given sedation or anesthetic to help you relax and reduce pain during the treatment. This may be administered via an IV line or as a throat spray.

4. Inserting the Endoscope: Once you are at ease, the doctor will gently introduce a thin, flexible tube known as an endoscope into your mouth and your esophagus, stomach, and, in some cases, the top section of your small intestine. The endoscope has a light and a camera, which allows the doctor to view your digestive system.

5. Examining the Digestive Tract: As the endoscope moves through your digestive system, the doctor will carefully check the linings of your esophagus, stomach, and duodenum.

They may collect tissue samples (biopsies) for additional examination if required.

6. Monitoring and Documentation: Throughout the process, the medical team will monitor your vital signs as well as the pictures obtained by the endoscope. They will record any anomalies or results that may need additional investigation or treatment.

7. After the examination, the doctor will gently remove the endoscope from your digestive system. You may feel slight pain or gagging while it is removed.

8. Recovery and Post-Procedure Care: Following the gastroscopy, you will be transferred to a recovery area to relax while the anesthetic wears off. Your doctor will go over the results with you and provide you with any required recommendations for post-procedure care or follow-up consultations.

Role Of The Endoscope

The endoscope is the principal instrument used in gastroscopy, enabling clinicians to see within the upper digestive tract. It comprises of a long, flexible tube with a light source and a small camera at the tip. Here's how the endoscope works and what its purpose is throughout the procedure:

1. Flexible and maneuverable: One of the endoscope's important qualities is its flexibility, which enables it to negotiate the twists and turns of the digestive system while causing the patient minimum pain. The doctor may direct the movement of the endoscope to get clear pictures of various places.

2. Illumination and Visualization: The endoscope has a strong light source that illuminates the esophagus, stomach, and duodenum. The camera at the tip takes high-definition photos in real time, giving comprehensive views of any anomalies including inflammation, ulcers, or tumors.

3. Biopsy Capability: In addition to visual assessment, the endoscope enables clinicians to conduct biopsies, which entail collecting tiny tissue samples for subsequent evaluation under a microscope. This is an important part of gastroscopy since it helps diagnose illnesses such as gastritis, esophagitis, and even some forms of cancer.

4. Endoscopes are available in a variety of sizes and designs to meet the diverse demands of patients and clinicians. Some endoscopes have suction and irrigation channels, as well as therapeutic devices for polyp excision or stent implantation.

5. Patient Comfort: While gastroscopy may seem daunting, the use of an endoscope usually relieves patients' suffering. The operation is normally conducted under sedation or anesthetic to help you relax and alleviate any gagging or pain caused by the endoscope insertion.

Anesthesia Options

Anesthesia is critical to maintaining the patient's comfort and compliance during gastroscopy. Depending on your medical history, preferences, and the intricacy of the treatment, your doctor may offer one of the following anesthetic options:

1. Conscious sedation, also known as twilight sedation, is the process of delivering drugs via an IV line to assist you relax and feeling sleepy throughout the treatment. You will be aware and able to react to orders, but your recall of the event may be limited.

2. **General Anesthesia:** If the gastroscopy is predicted to be extensive or if you have poor pain tolerance, your doctor may consider general anesthesia. This entails being completely asleep and unable to feel discomfort during the process. An anesthesiologist must closely watch the patient.

3. Local anesthetic may be utilized for individuals who want to be completely awake throughout the treatment, or if conscious sedation is not appropriate for medical reasons. Typically, a numbing drug is sprayed into the neck to alleviate pain during the endoscope insertion.

4. Patient Preferences: Your doctor will discuss the anesthetic alternatives with you beforehand, taking into account your preferences, medical history, and any possible dangers or contraindications. The objective is to keep you as comfortable as possible throughout the gastroscopy while ensuring safety and efficacy.

Possible Risks And Complications

While gastroscopy is usually considered a safe surgery, there are certain possible dangers and problems that you should be aware of:

1. Anesthesia Reaction: Some individuals may have adverse responses to anesthetic medicines, such as allergic reactions, respiratory depression, or cardiovascular issues. These dangers are usually greater with general anesthesia than with conscious sedation or local anesthesia.

2. Bleeding or Perforation: In rare situations, the insertion of the endoscope or the biopsy operation might result in bleeding or a rip in the digestive system. This might result in symptoms including stomach discomfort, bleeding, or infection, necessitating immediate medical intervention.

3. Infection: Although gastroscopy is conducted in a sterile environment, there is still a slight risk of infection, especially if the endoscope is not adequately cleansed and disinfected between treatments. This danger is reduced by adhering to stringent cleanliness measures and utilizing disposable attachments wherever feasible.

4. Pain and Complications: Some patients may have brief pain after the treatment, such as sore throat, bloating, or nausea. These symptoms often subside within a few hours to days. However, if you have chronic or severe symptoms, you should see your doctor for additional assessment.

5. Adverse responses: In rare cases, patients may develop adverse responses to the surgery itself, such as stomach contents aspiration (inhalation), allergic reactions to drugs or contrast agents used during the procedure, or cardiac events such as arrhythmias or heart attacks.

6. Follow-up Care: To reduce the risk of complications and ensure proper recovery, it is critical to adhere to any post-procedure instructions provided by your doctor, such as avoiding certain activities or medications, monitoring for signs of infection or bleeding, and attending follow-up appointments on schedule.

CHAPTER 4

The Gastroscopy Suite

Introduction To The Endoscopy Room

Welcome to the Gastroscopy Suite, where critical medical procedures are performed to diagnose and treat a variety of gastrointestinal problems. This customized facility is intended to allow gastroscopy, a technique in which a flexible tube with a camera is put via the mouth to study the upper digestive system.

The Endoscopy Room is precisely planned to guarantee the safety and comfort of both patients and medical personnel. As you go in, you'll see that it's a hygienic atmosphere, with equipment nicely organized and important instruments easily available. The chamber is outfitted with cutting-edge equipment that allows for precise and efficient gastroscopy procedures.

Equipment Used For Gastroscopy

Several critical pieces of equipment are utilized in the Gastroscopy Suite to ensure that the operation runs well. The gastroscope is the most visible instrument, a flexible tube outfitted with a camera and a light source. This technology enables the medical team to see the inner linings of the esophagus, stomach, and duodenum in real-time.

There is also a monitor linked to the gastroscope that displays high-definition pictures taken throughout the process. This enables the gastroenterologist to thoroughly inspect the digestive system and detect any abnormalities or lesions.

Other necessary equipment includes a suction device to remove excess saliva and fluids from the mouth during the process, as well as air and water channels inside the gastroscope to inflate the digestive system for improved visibility and clean the region as required.

Roles For Healthcare Professionals

The Gastroscopy Suite is manned by a diverse team of healthcare specialists, each of whom plays a critical part in assuring the procedure's success and the patient's safety.

The gastroenterologist is the main medical specialist responsible for carrying out the gastroscopy. They have had considerable endoscopic training and are proficient at using the gastroscope to safely travel the digestive system and properly interpret the results.

A team of nurses and technologists works with the gastroenterologist to assist in the process. They help prepare the patient, aid with positioning, and manage the equipment and supplies required for the gastroscopy. Their presence promotes seamless synchronization and increases patient comfort and safety.

Patient Comfort Measures

Patient comfort is a high focus in the Gastroscopy Suite, and many steps are taken to reduce pain and anxiety throughout the process.

Before the gastroscopy, patients are usually given a sedative or anesthesia to help them relax and alleviate any pain. The medical staff makes sure the patient is in a comfortable posture, generally resting on their side, and offers blankets or pillows for extra support.

Throughout the process, medical personnel converse with the patient, offering comfort and direction. Patients are taught to breathe gently and deeply to help them relax even more.

Following the gastroscopy, patients are constantly observed while they recover from sedation. The medical team gives the patient post-procedure care instructions and answers any concerns or questions they may have.

To summarize, the Gastroscopy Suite is a dedicated setting in which gastroscopy operations are carried out with accuracy, professionalism, and an emphasis on patient comfort. The devoted team of healthcare specialists and innovative technology guarantee that the treatment is carried out safely and properly, delivering significant information about the health of the upper digestive system.

CHAPTER 5

Patient Experiences During Gastroscopy

The Arrival And Registration Process

When patients arrive at the medical institution for a gastroscopy, they are met by receptionists who walk them through the registration procedure. This often entails disclosing personal information, medical history, and insurance information. The staff may also confirm the objective of the visit and ensure that any required documentation is completed. This first step attempts to simplify administrative processes and guarantee that patient data are correct and up to date.

After registering, patients are often required to remain in the designated waiting room until their surgery begins. During this time, patients may be given information about what to expect during the gastroscopy, such as specifics regarding the surgery, any risks or problems, and pre-procedure instructions.

During this waiting time, patients may mentally prepare and ask any last-minute queries.

Pre-Procedure Preparation In The Waiting Area

Patients may be instructed to prepare for their gastroscopy while they wait. This may require fasting for a certain length of time, often 6 to 8 hours, to ensure the stomach is empty. Fasting reduces the risk of problems during the surgery and allows for improved vision of the gastrointestinal system.

In addition to fasting, patients may need to avoid certain drugs or supplements before the operation since they may interfere with the results or raise the risk of bleeding. Before the gastroscopy, patients should strictly adhere to their healthcare provider's medication management guidelines.

During the pre-procedure preparation time, patients may be required to change into hospital gowns and remove any jewelry or accessories. This improves patient comfort and safety throughout the treatment and provides better access to the region under examination.

Transition To The Procedure Room

Once the patient is prepared for the gastroscopy, a healthcare practitioner or nurse will accompany them from the waiting area to the operation room. In the procedure room, the patient will meet the gastroenterologist who will do the examination, as well as any assistance personnel.

Before the treatment starts, the healthcare team will go over the patient's medical history, confirm any allergies or pre-existing diseases, and answer any concerns or questions the patient may have. This pre-procedure conversation ensures that the patient is completely educated and comfortable before beginning with the gastroscopy.

When the patient is ready, they will be pleasantly positioned on the examination table, usually lying on their left side. The healthcare team will next provide sedation, either by an intravenous (IV) line or oral medicine, to assist the patient in rest and reduce pain throughout the treatment.

Post-Operative Care And Recovery

Following the gastroscopy, patients are usually observed in a recovery area until they are completely awake and conscious. Sedation's effects might vary from person to person, thus patients should be monitored for any adverse reactions or consequences.

Patients may encounter modest side effects throughout their recuperation, such as bloating, gas, or a sore throat. These symptoms are often transient and should subside within a few hours.

Patients should avoid driving or using heavy equipment for the remainder of the day owing to the sedative effects.

Before discharge, patients will get post-procedure instructions from their healthcare practitioner, which may include food advice, medication restrictions, and any follow-up visits that may be required. Patients must carefully follow these guidelines to ensure a smooth recovery and the best possible results after their gastroscopy.

CHAPTER 6

Interpreting Gastroscopy Results

Explanation Of Gastroscopic Findings

A gastroscopy involves inserting a thin, flexible tube with a camera at the tip, known as an endoscope, through the mouth and down into the stomach and the beginning of the small intestine. This treatment enables physicians to see the lining of the digestive system and detect any abnormalities. The results of a gastroscopy may provide important information regarding the health of the upper gastrointestinal tract, which includes the esophagus, stomach, and intestine.

The gastroscopy results might vary based on the purpose of the surgery and the individual's health status. Inflammation, ulcers, tumors, polyps, bleeding, and infection are all common findings.

These results aid physicians in diagnosing different gastrointestinal problems and developing suitable treatment plans.

Inflammation defined as redness and swelling of the digestive system lining, might suggest illnesses such as gastritis, esophagitis, or duodenitis. Ulcers are open sores that form in the stomach or duodenal lining. They are often caused by Helicobacter pylori bacteria infection or long-term use of nonsteroidal anti-inflammatory medicines (NSAIDs). Tumors, both benign and malignant, may be discovered during gastroscopy and may need further assessment and treatment.

Polyps are tiny growths that may form on the inside lining of the digestive system. While most polyps are harmless, some may become cancerous over time. Identifying and eliminating polyps during gastroscopy may aid in the prevention of cancer.

Bleeding in the gastrointestinal system may appear as visible blood or as signs of recent bleeding, such as blood clots or black, tarry stools. Ulcers, inflammation, or rips in the esophageal or stomach lining are all potential causes of bleeding.

Gastroscopy may identify infections caused by Helicobacter pylori bacteria as well as the presence of fungal species such as Candida. Antibiotics or antifungal drugs may be required to remove the microorganisms and ease symptoms in these cases.

Common Conditions Detected

Gastroscopy is an effective diagnostic procedure for diagnosing a variety of gastrointestinal problems. Some of the most frequent conditions identified during a gastroscopy are:

1. Gastritis is an acute or chronic inflammation of the stomach lining that may be caused by infection, irritation, or autoimmune diseases.

2. Peptic Ulcers: Open sores on the stomach or duodenum's inner lining, most often caused by Helicobacter pylori infection or extended use of NSAIDs.

3. Esophagitis is esophageal inflammation that is most usually caused by acid reflux, infections, or certain drugs.

4. Barrett's Esophagus: A condition in which the cells that line the lower esophagus alter as a result of persistent acid reflux, increasing the chance of developing esophageal cancer.

5. Esophageal varices are enlarged veins in the lower esophageal walls that are often linked with liver illness and portal hypertension. If ruptured, they may cause significant bleeding.

6. Gastroesophageal Reflux Disease (GERD) is a chronic illness defined by the reflux of stomach acid into the esophagus, which causes symptoms such as heartburn and regurgitation.

7. Gastric cancer is a malignant tumor that develops in the stomach lining and might manifest as abnormal growths or ulcerated lesions during a gastroscopy.

Detecting these problems early via gastroscopy allows for timely treatment, which may help reduce complications and improve patient outcomes.

The Significance Of Biopsy Samples

During gastroscopy, the endoscopist may take biopsy samples from abnormal-looking sections of the digestive system to examine under a microscope. Biopsy samples are tiny tissue specimens that enable pathologists to analyze the cells and detect abnormalities such as inflammation, infection, or malignant growth.

Biopsy samples are critical for diagnosing and managing gastrointestinal illnesses. They give clear information regarding the type and severity of the underlying illness, which informs therapy choices and prognosis. For example, a biopsy revealing the presence of Helicobacter pylori bacteria may trigger the start of antibiotic treatment to clear the infection and avoid peptic ulcer recurrence.

In situations of suspected cancer, biopsy samples aid in determining the kind, stage, and aggressiveness of the tumor, allowing physicians to create individualized treatment regimens such as surgery, chemotherapy, or radiation therapy. Early identification of cancer by biopsy may considerably increase the likelihood of effective therapy and long-term survival.

Biopsy samples are often acquired by passing specialized devices, such as forceps or brushes, via the endoscope's working channel. The treatment is usually painless and requires no extra incisions or anesthetic. Following collection, biopsy specimens are submitted to a pathology facility for processing and examination.

Communicating Results To Patients

After conducting a gastroscopy and evaluating the findings, the gastroenterologist or endoscopist delivers the findings to the patient in a comprehensible way. Effective communication is critical for ensuring that patients understand their diagnosis, treatment choices, and prognosis, allowing them to make educated healthcare decisions.

During the discussion of gastroscopy results, the healthcare professional describes the findings in layman's words, avoiding medical jargon and utilizing visual aids like photos or diagrams to highlight crucial areas. They describe the importance of any abnormalities discovered, possible reasons, and suggested next actions, such as more testing or therapies.

The healthcare professional answers any questions or concerns made by the patient, offering comfort and assistance as required.

They also address lifestyle and nutritional adjustments that may help manage gastrointestinal diseases, such as avoiding spicy foods or alcohol in the case of gastritis or implementing dietary and behavioral changes to lessen acid reflux symptoms.

In situations when biopsy samples are collected during a gastroscopy, the healthcare professional discusses the purpose of the procedure, the possible hazards, and the significance of waiting for pathology findings before making final diagnoses or treatment plans.

Overall, efficient communication between healthcare practitioners and patients builds trust, increases patient satisfaction, and promotes treatment adherence, resulting in improved results in the management of gastrointestinal illnesses.

CHAPTER 7

Possible Complications And Safety Measures

Common Complications During Gastroscopy

Gastroscopy, like any other medical treatment, has certain dangers, although they are typically low. One typical hazard is a response to the sedative used during the surgery. While it is uncommon, some people may develop allergic responses or side effects such as nausea, vomiting, or dizziness. To reduce this danger, your healthcare practitioner will first analyze your medical history and allergies and alter the sedative appropriately.

Another possible consequence is bleeding. During gastroscopy, a biopsy may be performed to further investigate any abnormalities seen in the digestive system. In rare situations, the biopsy site may bleed after the operation. However, your doctor will constantly watch you for any indications of bleeding and take fast action if required.

Perforation, or puncture of the digestive system, is a very uncommon but significant consequence of gastroscopy. This might happen if there is too much force used during the surgery or if there are pre-existing disorders that weaken the digestive system wall. Perforation symptoms include severe stomach discomfort, fever, and trouble breathing. If detected, get quick medical assistance to avoid additional consequences.

Emergency Procedures For Complications

In the case of difficulties during or after a gastroscopy, healthcare personnel are trained to act quickly and efficiently to protect patient safety. If a patient has an unfavorable response to the sedative, healthcare personnel will constantly monitor their vital signs and prescribe drugs to counteract the effects. In extreme circumstances, they may need to provide breathing assistance or other procedures to help stabilize the patient.

If bleeding develops during or after a gastroscopy, healthcare practitioners will take action to stop it, such as applying pressure to the biopsy site or providing clotting agents. In rare situations of severe bleeding, further treatments such as endoscopic therapy or surgery may be required to halt the bleeding and avoid consequences.

In the uncommon case of a perforation, prompt surgical intervention is essential to heal the hole and avoid infection. Healthcare personnel will carefully monitor the patient for symptoms of sepsis or other problems and will provide appropriate therapy as required.

Healthcare Providers Follow Safety Protocols

Healthcare practitioners adhere to stringent safety standards to reduce the risk of problems during gastroscopy. To guarantee the safest possible experience, patients are evaluated thoroughly before the surgery, including their medical history, current medicines, and any allergies.

To avoid infections, healthcare personnel employ sterile equipment and aseptic practices throughout the treatment. They also carefully monitor vital signs and react quickly to any changes in the patient's condition.

Following the treatment, patients are carefully observed in a recovery room until the sedation wears off and they are declared stable enough to be discharged. Patients are given guidelines for post-procedure care and are urged to contact their doctor if they have any unexpected symptoms or consequences.

Patients' Rights And Advocacy

As a patient undergoing gastroscopy, you have rights and duties that healthcare practitioners must uphold. You have the right to be informed about the procedure, including its risks and benefits, and to agree to or reject treatment based on that knowledge.

You also have the right to privacy and secrecy throughout the process, as well as the option to have a support person present if necessary. If you have any concerns or questions concerning the surgery, please address them with your healthcare professional beforehand.

Advocacy is critical to preserving patient safety and providing high-quality treatment during gastroscopy. If you have any concerns about the treatment or the care you get, you should speak out and advocate for yourself. You may ask questions, get clarification, or request more information to ensure that you understand what to anticipate and that your requirements are addressed.

Being proactive and involved in your healthcare may help guarantee a great experience and reduce the chance of problems during a gastroscopy. Your healthcare team is here to help you every step of the way, so please do not hesitate to contact us if you have any issues or questions.

CHAPTER 8

Lifestyle Changes And Follow-Up Care

Dietary And Lifestyle Recommendations Following Gastroscopy

After a gastroscopy, you need to make certain changes to your diet and lifestyle to promote optimum healing and avoid problems. Here's a detailed guide on what dietary and lifestyle adjustments you may need to make:

Dietary recommendations:

1. Soft meals: To allow your digestive system to recuperate, start with soft, easily digested meals. Soups, yogurt, mashed potatoes, and smoothies may be easy on the stomach.

2. Avoid Spicy and Acidic Meals: Spicy meals, as well as acidic and citrusy foods such as tomatoes and oranges, might irritate the stomach lining.

3. Gradual Reintroduction of Solid Meals: Once you're feeling better, gradually resume eating solid meals. Begin with mild foods such as rice, boiled chicken, and toast before progressing to bigger meals.

4. Hydration: Drink lots of water to keep hydrated, particularly if you suffer vomiting or diarrhea after the surgery. Dehydration may delay the healing process.

5. Limit Alcohol and Caffeine: Avoid alcohol and caffeine for a few days after gastroscopy since they may irritate the stomach lining and interfere with healing.

Lifestyle recommendations:

1. Relax and Relaxation: Allow yourself time to relax and recuperate after the treatment. Avoid intense activity for a day or two to enable your body to fully recuperate.

2. Medication Management: Follow your doctor's recommendations for any medicines you may need to take after gastroscopy. Avoid NSAIDs (nonsteroidal anti-inflammatory medicines), such as ibuprofen, since they might raise the risk of bleeding.

3. Quit Smoking: If you are a smoker, try quitting or lowering your smoking habits. Smoking may slow recovery and raise the risk of problems.

4. Stress Management: Stress may aggravate gastrointestinal problems, so use stress-reduction practices such as deep breathing, meditation, or yoga to assist recovery.

5. Follow-up with Your Doctor: Make all planned follow-up visits with your doctor to track your progress and handle any concerns or issues that may occur.

Following these dietary and lifestyle suggestions can help your body recover and reduce the risk of problems after a gastroscopy.

The Importance Of Follow-Up Appointments

Follow-up consultations following a gastroscopy are critical for tracking your progress, resolving issues, and maintaining long-term health. Here's why these appointments are important:

1. Monitoring recovery: Your doctor will examine how well your stomach and esophagus are recovering after the surgery. They will search for symptoms of inflammation, ulcers, or other issues that may need further therapy.

2. Adjusting Treatment: If any anomalies are discovered during the gastroscopy, follow-up sessions enable your doctor to modify your treatment plan appropriately. This might include beginning or changing medicines, suggesting lifestyle modifications, or arranging further testing or procedures.

3. Preventing problems: Early identification and care may help avoid problems including bleeding, infection, or gastrointestinal recurrence. Follow-up visits help your doctor to identify any possible issues before they worsen.

4. Addressing Concerns: If you notice any new symptoms or side effects after your gastroscopy, your follow-up visit is a chance to address them with your doctor. They may advice on how to manage these symptoms and give comfort if necessary.

5. Long-term Management: Gastrointestinal problems often need long-term treatment and monitoring. Follow-up consultations assist in building a plan for continuing treatment and verify that you're getting the support you need to keep your digestive system healthy.

General, attending follow-up visits is critical for improving the result of your gastroscopy and ensuring your general health.

Monitor For Recurrence Or New Symptoms

Following a gastroscopy, it is critical to monitor for any indications of recurrence or new symptoms that might suggest underlying gastrointestinal problems. Here's what to look out for:

1. **Persistent Symptoms:** If you continue to have symptoms such as stomach discomfort, bloating, nausea, vomiting, or trouble swallowing following the gastroscopy, it may suggest an unsolved problem that requires additional investigation.

2. **Changes in Symptoms:** Be aware of any changes in the frequency, intensity, or character of your symptoms.

New or worsening symptoms might suggest a relapse of the underlying ailment or the emergence of a new issue.

3. **Bleeding:** Call your doctor right away if you notice any indications of bleeding, such as black or bloody stools, vomiting blood, or feeling lightheaded or dizzy.

These might be symptoms of a problem that needs immediate medical intervention.

4. Persistent tiredness: Chronic tiredness or weakness may suggest anemia, which is caused by gastrointestinal bleeding. If you feel particularly fatigued or weak, especially if it is accompanied by additional symptoms such as pale skin or shortness of breath, get medical help right once.

5. Significant and unexplained weight loss may indicate underlying gastrointestinal disorders such as malabsorption, inflammation, or malignancy. If you observe a rapid or sustained weight loss without attempting, see your doctor.

It is important to swiftly convey any new or worrying symptoms to your healthcare practitioner so that they can identify the best course of action, whether it be more testing, medication adjustments, or lifestyle changes.

When To Seek Medical Attention?

While some pain and mild symptoms are usual after a gastroscopy, other signals need rapid medical treatment. Here are some scenarios in which you should seek immediate medical attention:

1. Significant stomach Pain: If you have significant stomach pain that does not go away with over-the-counter pain medicines or that continues after rest, it might be due to a complication like perforation or bleeding.

2. Difficulty breathing or shortness of breath may indicate a significant consequence, such as aspiration pneumonia or a sedative response. If you're having difficulties breathing, get medical help immediately.

3. A temperature of more than 100.4°F (38°C) with chills or sweating may suggest an illness. If you get a fever after the surgery, contact your doctor.

4. Persistent Vomiting: Constant vomiting, particularly if it includes blood or resembles coffee grounds, may suggest a problem such as hemorrhage or stomach perforation. Seek medical care right now.

5. Shock symptoms include a fast pulse, short breathing, cold or clammy skin, and disorientation, which may be life-threatening and need emergency medical attention. If you or someone else is showing indications of shock, contact emergency services.

If you're worried about any symptoms or changes in your health, you should follow your instincts and seek medical attention. Prompt action may assist to avoid significant problems and provide the best possible result.

CHAPTER 9

Gastroscopy In Special Populations

Gastroscopy For Children And Infants

Gastroscopy in children and babies needs extra attention and care owing to their tiny stature and specific physiological requirements. The surgery is often conducted under general anesthesia to keep the youngster quiet and comfortable throughout. Before the surgery, the kid may be instructed to fast for a certain length of time to ensure that the stomach is empty and reduce the chance of aspiration during anesthesia.

During the gastroscopy, a pediatric endoscope with a smaller diameter is utilized to inspect the esophagus, stomach, and duodenum. The treatment is normally quick, lasting between 15 and 30 minutes. Parents may be permitted to accompany their children to give comfort and support during the procedure.

Following the gastroscopy, the kid may have moderate pain or bloating, which normally resolves rapidly. Parents must follow any post-procedure recommendations given by healthcare professionals, such as cautiously restarting feeding and watching for symptoms of problems.

Gastroscopy For Elderly Patients

Gastroscopy in older adults necessitates a detailed assessment of their general health and any underlying medical issues. Older persons may be more vulnerable to problems such as aspiration or cardiovascular events during the treatment, thus a complete pre-procedure examination is required.

The gastroscopy operation is identical to that used in younger individuals, but extra measures may be used to protect the safety and comfort of older patients. This might entail carefully monitoring vital signs throughout the surgery and delivering supplementary oxygen if required.

Following the gastroscopy, older people may take longer to recover and may suffer weariness or sleepiness. During the healing time, caregivers must offer support and help as required, as well as keep an eye out for indicators of problems such as bleeding or infection.

Considerations For Pregnant Women

Gastroscopy is typically safe for pregnant women, but some care should be followed to reduce possible dangers to both the mother and the baby. The treatment is normally carried out during the second trimester when the risk of problems is lowest.

Before the gastroscopy, the healthcare team will evaluate the procedure's possible advantages and hazards for both the mother and the fetus.

Alternative imaging procedures may be used if the dangers of gastroscopy are regarded as too great.

During the gastroscopy, the mother's vital signs and oxygen levels are continuously checked to assure her and the fetus' safety. The operation is identical to that performed on non-pregnant patients, although the healthcare team may take additional precautions to reduce the mother's pain or worry.

Adapting Gastroscopy To Patients With Specific Medical Conditions

Gastroscopy may be customized to treat individuals with particular medical disorders, including swallowing problems or anatomical anomalies. In certain circumstances, specialist equipment or procedures may be used to guarantee a successful treatment.

Patients with esophageal strictures or constriction may need dilatation before gastroscopy to enable the endoscope to pass through safely. Similarly, individuals with anatomical differences, such as hiatal hernias, may need different placement during the treatment to improve visibility.

The healthcare staff will carefully consider each patient's specific requirements and modify the gastroscopy operation appropriately. This might include pre-procedure testing or meetings with other professionals to guarantee the safest and most effective method.

What To Expect During And After A Gastroscopy

To promote patient comfort and compliance during a gastroscopy surgery, sedation or anesthesia is usually used. The endoscope is then inserted via the mouth into the esophagus, stomach, and duodenum, enabling the healthcare professional to carefully inspect these tissues.

Patients may suffer pain or gagging during the treatment, however this is typically tolerable owing to the effects of anesthesia. Patients may have bloating or a sore throat after the gastroscopy, although these symptoms usually pass within a few hours.

In rare situations, the healthcare professional may conduct biopsies or other procedures during the gastroscopy operation. Patients will be advised of any extra procedures or follow-up treatment that may be required depending on the results of the gastroscopy.

Addressing Anxiety And Apprehension

It is normal for people to feel frightened or hesitant about having a gastroscopy, particularly if it is their first time. However, it is important to note that gastroscopy is a normal and typically safe surgery conducted by skilled healthcare professionals.

To assist reduce anxiety, patients should ask their healthcare professional any questions they may have regarding the surgery ahead of time. It may also be beneficial to understand more about what to anticipate during the gastroscopy and how to prepare, including any fasting or medication requirements.

Patients may relax throughout the operation by focusing on deep breathing or using visualization methods. The healthcare staff will also make every effort to guarantee the patient's comfort and address any worries or discomfort that may arise throughout the treatment.

Following the gastroscopy, patients should follow any post-procedure advice offered by the healthcare team, including rest and food restrictions as needed. If patients have any concerns or have unexpected symptoms after the surgery, they should contact their healthcare practitioner for more information and assistance.

CHAPTER 10

Progress In Gastroscopy And Future Prospects

Emerging Technologies In Gastrointestinal Endoscopy

Gastrointestinal endoscopy technology has advanced significantly, making it more effective, efficient, and patient-friendly. One of the most important advancements is the development of high-definition imaging systems, which allow for crisper and more comprehensive images of the digestive tract. These devices combine modern optics and image processing techniques to improve visibility, enabling doctors to spot anomalies more accurately.

Another ground-breaking technique is narrow-band imaging (NBI), which uses certain wavelengths of light to improve contrast between various tissues in the gastrointestinal system. NBI increases lesion delineation and early-stage cancer diagnosis. By emphasizing tiny changes in tissue architecture, NBI enables gastroenterologists to make more exact diagnoses and guide focused therapies.

Furthermore, the use of artificial intelligence (AI) in gastroscopy has the potential to transform the area. AI systems can evaluate endoscopic pictures in real-time, helping physicians spot irregularities, forecast illness development, and even offer the best treatment choices. This technology shows potential for increasing diagnostic accuracy, shortening procedure times, and improving overall patient care.

Potential Areas Of Research And Innovation

As gastroscopy evolves, researchers are looking for new ways to enhance and innovate. One area of research is the development of smaller endoscopic equipment that can reach further into the gastrointestinal system while causing minimum pain to the patient. These gadgets may include characteristics like wireless connection, robotic navigation, and enhanced imaging capabilities to improve diagnostic and therapeutic skills.

Furthermore, there is a rising interest in using molecular imaging methods for early identification of gastrointestinal illnesses. Fluorescence endoscopy and confocal laser endomicroscopy are two techniques that provide real-time observation of cellular and molecular changes, allowing for the early diagnosis of malignant or precancerous tumors. These tools, which identify anomalies at the molecular level, show promise for boosting screening accuracy and directing individualized treatment approaches.

Researchers are also investigating the possibilities of non-invasive imaging technologies like virtual colonoscopy and capsule endoscopy as alternatives to conventional gastroscopy. These approaches use modern imaging technology to see the gastrointestinal system without requiring invasive treatments. While still in the early phases of research, these non-invasive techniques have the potential to increase patient comfort and adherence to screening recommendations.

Improvements In Patient Experience And Safety

Advances in gastroscopy technology have resulted in major improvements to patient comfort and safety. Modern endoscopic systems include high-definition displays, ergonomic design, and better mobility, which enhance the comfort and safety of both patients and endoscopists. Furthermore, the use of sedation and anesthetic procedures suited to specific patient requirements reduces pain and anxiety during the surgery.

Furthermore, advances in infection control techniques have decreased the possibility of cross-contamination and infection transmission during gastroscopy.

Strict adherence to sterile protocols, complete washing and disinfection of endoscopic equipment, and careful handling of biological material all help to provide a safe and sanitary environment for patients having gastrointestinal operations.

The Changing Role Of Gastroscopy In Healthcare

Gastroscopy is essential in the diagnosis and treatment of a broad variety of gastrointestinal diseases, including reflux disease, peptic ulcers, colorectal cancer, and inflammatory bowel disease. As technology advances, the spectrum of gastroscopy applications grows, with new indications and procedures emerging regularly.

In addition to diagnostic purposes, gastroscopy is increasingly being utilized for therapeutic procedures such as polypectomy, mucosal resection, and stent insertion. These minimally invasive techniques provide excellent therapy for patients with gastrointestinal cancer, strictures, and other structural problems.

Furthermore, gastroscopy is essential in population-based screening programs for gastrointestinal malignancies, allowing for early diagnosis and management in high-risk patients. Gastroscopy, by detecting precancerous lesions and early-stage cancers, may considerably improve patient outcomes and minimize the burden of gastrointestinal malignancies on healthcare systems.

Overall, the future of gastroscopy seems promising, with continued advances in technology, research, and clinical practice positioned to improve its diagnostic and therapeutic capacities. By adopting these advancements and refining best practices, gastroenterologists may give the best possible treatment to patients suffering from a variety of gastrointestinal disorders.

Conclusion

In conclusion, knowing gastroscopy is critical for both patients and healthcare practitioners. This diagnostic method is critical for diagnosing and managing a variety of gastrointestinal diseases. Gastroscopy, which uses a flexible endoscope, enables a thorough inspection of the upper digestive system, including the esophagus, stomach, and duodenum.

Throughout this tutorial, we've discussed gastroscopy's purpose, process, preparation, dangers, and advantages. We discovered that gastroscopy is often used to assess symptoms including stomach discomfort, trouble swallowing, and gastrointestinal bleeding. It may also help discover and evaluate problems including GERD, ulcers, tumors, and inflammation.

Fasting for a certain length of time before the procedure and according to the healthcare provider's particular instructions are common preparations for gastroscopy. This enables good visibility and lowers the likelihood of difficulties during the test. Patients having gastroscopy should be informed of the hazards, which include bleeding, perforation, and bad sedative responses, albeit these are infrequent.

Despite the dangers, the advantages of gastroscopy often surpass any possible consequences. Early identification and diagnosis of gastrointestinal problems using gastroscopy may result in more prompt therapeutic interventions, improved results, and a higher quality of life for patients. Furthermore, gastroscopy enables the conduct of treatments such as biopsies, polypectomies, and the removal of foreign items, which contribute to holistic patient care.

For healthcare personnel, a complete grasp of gastroscopy is required to execute the surgery safely and efficiently. Proper training, adherence to set protocols, and continuing quality assurance methods are essential for achieving optimum results and patient satisfaction. Furthermore, adequate communication with patients about the treatment, its goal, and any potential dangers or discomforts is critical for establishing trust and reducing fear.

In conclusion, gastroscopy is an important technique in the diagnosis and treatment of gastrointestinal disorders. Gastroscopy, which provides a comprehensive inspection of the upper digestive system, aids in the diagnosis of problems, directing treatment options, and improving patient outcomes. Gastroscopy may be conducted safely and quickly with participation from patients, healthcare professionals, and support workers, improving overall gastrointestinal care quality.

THE END

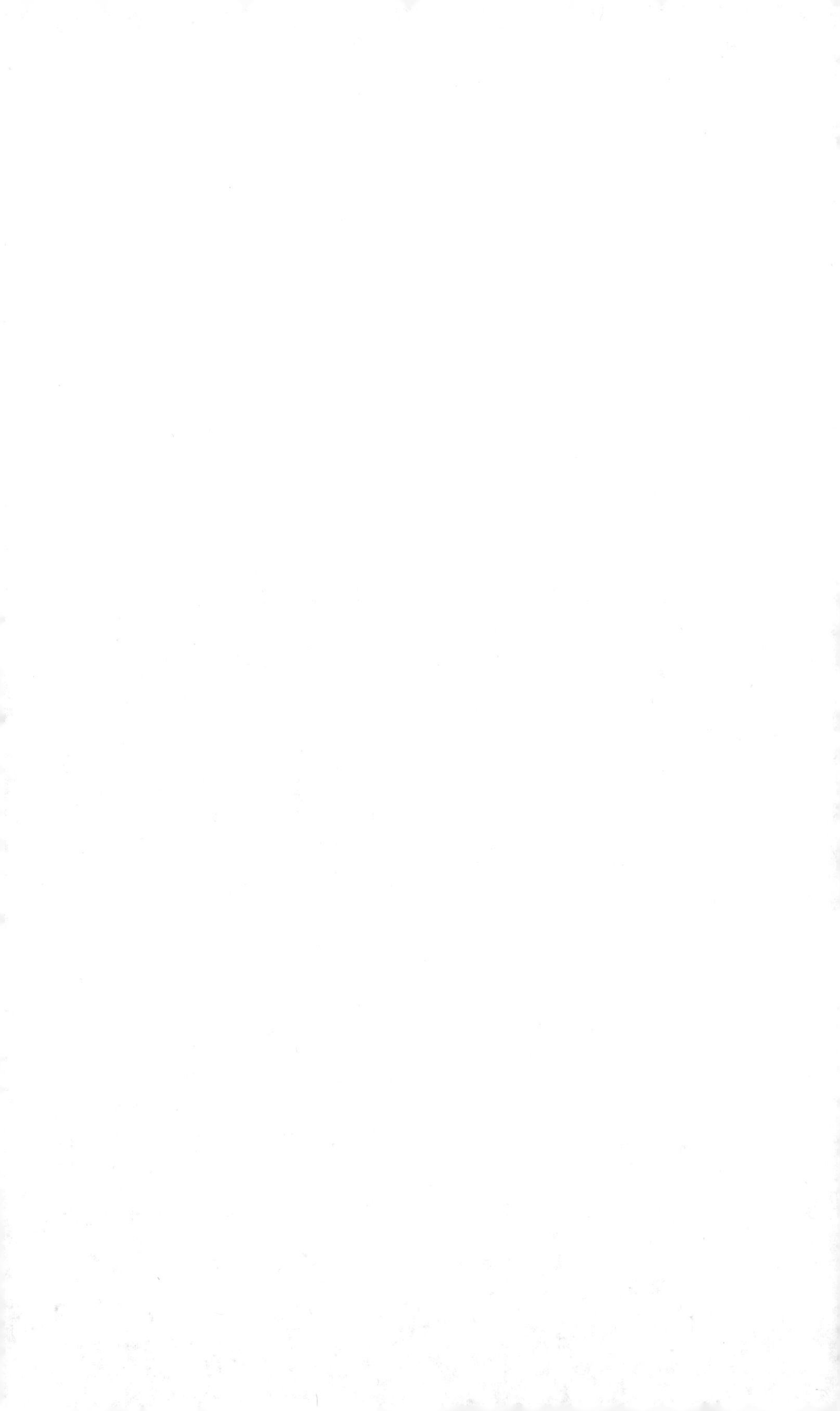

www.ingramcontent.com/pod-product-compliance
Lightning Source LLC
Chambersburg PA
CBHW051907250726
48659CB00002B/519